The Best Mediterranean Dash Diet Recipe Book

A Set of Mouth-Watering Recipes for Delicious Mediterranean Dash Diet Meals

Kathyrn Solano

By reading this document, the reader agrees that under no circumstances is the author responsible for any losses, direct or indirect, which are incurred as a result of the use of information contained within this document, including, but not limited to, — errors, omissions, or inaccuracies.

Table of contents

MEAT RECIPES

Authentic Aioli Baked Chicken Wings

Servings: 4

Cooking Time: 35 Minutes

Ingredients:

4 chicken wings

1 cup Halloumi cheese, cubed

1 tablespoon garlic, finely minced

1 tablespoon fresh lime juice

1 tablespoon fresh coriander, chopped

6 black olives, pitted and halved

1 ½ tablespoons butter

1 hard-boiled egg yolk

1 tablespoon balsamic vinegar

1/2 cup extra-virgin olive oil

1/4 teaspoon flaky sea salt

Sea salt and pepper, to season

Directions:

In a saucepan, melt the butter until sizzling. Sear the chicken wings for 5 minutes per side. Season with salt and pepper to taste.

Place the chicken wings on a parchment-lined baking pan

Mix the egg yolk, garlic, lime juice, balsamic vinegar, olive oil, and salt in your blender until creamy, uniform and smooth.

Spread the Aioli over the fried chicken. Now, scatter the coriander and black olives on top of the chicken wings.

Bake in the preheated oven at 380 degrees F for 20 to 2minutes.

Top with the cheese and bake an additional 5 minutes until hot and bubbly.

Storing

Place the chicken wings in airtight containers or Ziploc bags; keep in your refrigerator for up 3 to 4 days.

For freezing, place the chicken wings in airtight containers or heavy-duty freezer bags. Freeze up to 3 months. Once thawed in the refrigerator, heat in the preheated oven at 375 degrees F for 20 to 25 minutes or until heated through. Enjoy!

Nutrition Info: 562 Calories; 43.8g Fat; 2.1g Carbs; 40.8g Protein; 0.4g Fiber

Smoked Pork Sausage Keto Bombs

Servings: 6

Cooking Time: 15 Minutes

Ingredients:

3/4 pound smoked pork sausage, ground

1 teaspoon ginger-garlic paste

2 tablespoons scallions, minced

1 tablespoon butter, room temperature

1 tomato, pureed

4 ounces mozzarella cheese, crumbled

2 tablespoons flaxseed meal

8 ounces cream cheese, room temperature

Sea salt and ground black pepper, to taste

Directions:

Melt the butter in a frying pan over medium-high heat. Cook the sausage for about 4 minutes, crumbling with a spatula.

Add in the ginger-garlic paste, scallions, and tomato; continue to cook over medium-low heat for a further 6 minutes. Stir in the remaining ingredients.

Place the mixture in your refrigerator for 1 to 2 hours until firm.

Roll the mixture into bite-sized balls.

Storing

Transfer the balls to the airtight containers and place in your refrigerator for up to 3 days.

For freezing, place in a freezer safe containers and freeze up to 1 month. Enjoy!

Nutrition Info: 383 Calories; 32. Fat; 5.1g Carbs; 16.7g Protein; 1.7g Fiber

Turkey Meatballs With Tangy Basil Chutney

Servings: 6

Cooking Time: 30 Minutes

Ingredients:

2 tablespoons sesame oil

For the Meatballs:

1/2 cup Romano cheese, grated

1 teaspoon garlic, minced

1/2 teaspoon shallot powder

1/4 teaspoon dried thyme

1/2 teaspoon mustard seeds

2 small-sized eggs, lightly beaten

1 ½ pounds ground turkey

1/2 teaspoon sea salt

1/4 teaspoon ground black pepper, or more to taste

3 tablespoons almond meal

For the Basil Chutney:

2 tablespoons fresh lime juice

1/4 cup fresh basil leaves

1/4 cup fresh parsley

1/2 cup cilantro leaves

1 teaspoon fresh ginger root, grated

2 tablespoons olive oil

2 tablespoons water

1 tablespoon habanero chili pepper, deveined and minced

Directions:

In a mixing bowl, combine all ingredients for the meatballs. Roll the mixture into meatballs and reserve.

Heat the sesame oil in a frying pan over a moderate flame. Sear the meatballs for about 8 minutes until browned on all sides.

Make the chutney by mixing all the ingredients in your blender or food processor.

Storing

Place the meatballs in airtight containers or Ziploc bags; keep in your refrigerator for up to 3 to 4 days.

Freeze the meatballs in airtight containers or heavy-duty freezer bags. Freeze up to 3 to 4 months. To defrost, slowly reheat in a frying pan.

Store the basil chutney in the refrigerator for up to a week. Bon appétit!

Nutrition Info: 390 Calories; 27.2g Fat; 1. Carbs; 37.4g Protein; 0.3g Fiber

Roasted Chicken With Cashew Pesto

Servings: 4

Cooking Time: 35 Minutes

Ingredients:

1 cup leeks, chopped

1 pound chicken legs, skinless

Salt and ground black pepper, to taste

1/2 teaspoon red pepper flakes

For the Cashew-Basil Pesto:

1/2 cup cashews

2 garlic cloves, minced

1/2 cup fresh basil leaves

1/2 cup Parmigiano-Reggiano cheese, preferably freshly grated

1/2 cup olive oil

Directions:

Place the chicken legs in a parchment-lined baking pan. Season with salt and pepper, Then, scatter the leeks around the chicken legs.

Roast in the preheated oven at 390 degrees F for 30 to 35 minutes, rotating the pan occasionally.

Pulse the cashews, basil, garlic, and cheese in your blender until pieces are small. Continue blending while adding olive oil to the mixture. Mix until the desired consistency is reached.

Storing

Place the chicken in airtight containers or Ziploc bags; keep in your refrigerator for up 3 to 4 days.

To freeze the chicken legs, place them in airtight containers or heavy-duty freezer bags. Freeze up to 3 months. Once thawed in the refrigerator, heat in the preheated oven at 375 degrees F for 20 to 25 minutes.

Store your pesto in the refrigerator for up to a week. Bon appétit!

Nutrition Info: 5 Calories; 44.8g Fat; 5g Carbs; 38.7g Protein; 1g Fiber

Duck Breasts In Boozy Sauce

Servings: 4

Cooking Time: 20 Minutes

Ingredients:

1 ½ pounds duck breasts, butterflied

1 tablespoon tallow, room temperature

1 ½ cups chicken consommé

3 tablespoons soy sauce

2 ounces vodka

1/2 cup sour cream

4 scallion stalks, chopped

Salt and pepper, to taste

Directions:

Melt the tallow in a frying pan over medium-high flame. Sear the duck breasts for about 5 minutes, flipping them over occasionally to ensure even cooking.

Add in the scallions, salt, pepper, chicken consommé, and soy sauce. Partially cover and continue to cook for a further 8 minutes.

Add in the vodka and sour cream; remove from the heat and stir to combine well.

Storing

Place the duck breasts in airtight containers or Ziploc bags; keep in your refrigerator for up to 3 to 4 days.

For freezing, place duck breasts in airtight containers or heavy-duty freezer bags. Freeze up to 2 to 3 months. Once thawed in the refrigerator, reheat in a saucepan. Bon appétit!

Nutrition Info: 351 Calories; 24. Fat; 6.6g Carbs; 22.1g Protein; 0.6g Fiber

White Cauliflower And Chicken Chowder

Servings: 6

Cooking Time: 30 Minutes

Ingredients:

1 cup leftover roast chicken breasts

1 head cauliflower, broken into small-sized florets

Sea salt and ground white pepper, to taste

2 ½ cups water

3 cups chicken consommé

1 ¼ cups sour cream

1/2 stick butter

1/2 cup white onion, finely chopped

1 teaspoon fresh garlic, finely minced

1 celery, chopped

Directions:

In a heavy bottomed pot, melt the butter over a moderate heat. Cook the onion, garlic and celery for about 5 minutes or until they've softened.

Add in the salt, white pepper, water, chicken consommé, chicken, and cauliflower florets; bring to a boil. Reduce the temperature to simmer and continue to cook for 30 minutes.

Puree the soup with an immersion blender. Fold in sour cream and stir to combine well.

Storing

Spoon your chowder into airtight containers or Ziploc bags; keep in your refrigerator for up to 3 to 4 days.

For freezing, place your chowder in airtight containers. It will maintain the best quality for about 4 to months. Defrost in the refrigerator. Bon appétit!

Nutrition Info: 231 Calories; 18.2g Fat; 5.9g Carbs; 11.9g Protein; 1.4g Fiber

Taro Leaf And Chicken Soup

Servings: 4

Cooking Time: 45 Minutes

Ingredients:

1 pound whole chicken, boneless and chopped into small chunks

1/2 cup onions, chopped

1/2 cup rutabaga, cubed

2 carrots, peeled

2 celery stalks

Salt and black pepper, to taste

1 cup chicken bone broth

1/2 teaspoon ginger-garlic paste

1/2 cup taro leaves, roughly chopped

1 tablespoon fresh coriander, chopped

3 cups water

1 teaspoon paprika

Directions:

Place all ingredients in a heavy-bottomed pot. Bring to a boil over the highest heat.

Turn the heat to simmer. Continue to cook, partially covered, an additional 40 minutes.

Storing

Spoon the soup into four airtight containers or Ziploc bags; keep in your refrigerator for up to 3 to days.

For freezing, place the soup in airtight containers. It will maintain the best quality for about to 6 months. Defrost in the refrigerator. Bon appétit!

Nutrition Info: 25Calories; 12.9g Fat; 3.2g Carbs; 35.1g Protein; 2.2g Fiber

Creamed Greek-style Soup

Servings: 4

Cooking Time: 30 Minutes

Ingredients:

1/2 stick butter

1/2 cup zucchini, diced

2 garlic cloves, minced

4 ½ cups roasted vegetable broth

Sea salt and ground black pepper, to season

1 ½ cups leftover turkey, shredded

1/3 cup double cream

1/2 cup Greek-style yogurt

Directions:

In a heavy-bottomed pot, melt the butter over medium-high heat. Once hot, cook the zucchini and garlic for 2 minutes until they are fragrant.

Add in the broth, salt, black pepper, and leftover turkey. Cover and cook for minutes, stirring periodically.

Then, fold in the cream and yogurt. Continue to cook for 5 minutes more or until thoroughly warmed.

Storing

Spoon the soup into four airtight containers or Ziploc bags; keep in your refrigerator for up to 3 to 4 days.

For freezing, place the soup in airtight containers. It will maintain the best quality for about 4 to months. Defrost in the refrigerator. Enjoy!

Nutrition Info: 256 Calories; 18.8g Fat; 5.4g Carbs; 15.8g Protein; 0.2g Fiber

Keto Pork Wraps

Servings: 4

Cooking Time: 15 Minutes

Ingredients:

1 pound ground pork

2 garlic cloves, finely minced

1 chili pepper, deveined and finely minced

1 teaspoon mustard powder

1 tablespoon sunflower seeds

2 tablespoons champagne vinegar

1 tablespoon coconut aminos

Celery salt and ground black pepper, to taste

2 scallion stalks, sliced

1 head lettuce

Directions:

Sear the ground pork in the preheated pan for about 8 minutes. Stir in the garlic, chili pepper, mustard seeds, and sunflower seeds; continue to sauté for minute longer or until aromatic.

Add in the vinegar, coconut aminos, salt, black pepper, and scallions. Stir to combine well.

Storing

Place the ground pork mixture in airtight containers or Ziploc bags; keep in your refrigerator for up to 3 to days.

For freezing, place the ground pork mixture it in airtight containers or heavy-duty freezer bags. Freeze up to 2 to 3 months. Defrost in the refrigerator and reheat in the skillet.

Add spoonfuls of the pork mixture to the lettuce leaves, wrap them and serve.

Nutrition Info: 281 Calories; 19.4g Fat; 5.1g Carbs; 22.1g Protein; 1.3g Fiber

Ground Pork Skillet

Servings: 4

Cooking Time: 25 Minutes

Ingredients:

1 ½ pounds ground pork

2 tablespoons olive oil

1 bunch kale, trimmed and roughly chopped

1 cup onions, sliced

1/4 teaspoon black pepper, or more to taste

1/4 cup tomato puree

1 bell pepper, chopped

1 teaspoon sea salt

1 cup chicken bone broth

1/4 cup port wine

2 cloves garlic, pressed

1 chili pepper, sliced

Directions:

Heat tablespoon of the olive oil in a cast-iron skillet over a moderately high heat. Now, sauté the onion, garlic, and peppers until they are tender and fragrant; reserve.

Heat the remaining tablespoon of olive oil; once hot, cook the ground pork and approximately 5 minutes until no longer pink.

Add in the other ingredients and continue to cook for 15 to 17 minutes or until cooked through.

Storing

Place the ground pork mixture in airtight containers or Ziploc bags; keep in your refrigerator for up to 3 to 4 days.

For freezing, place the ground pork mixture in airtight containers or heavy-duty freezer bags. Freeze up to 2 to 3 months. Defrost in the refrigerator. Bon appétit!

Nutrition Info: 349 Calories; 13g Fat; 4.4g Carbs; 45.3g Protein; 1.2g Fiber

Cheesy Chinese-style Pork

Servings: 6

Cooking Time: 20 Minutes

Ingredients:

1 tablespoon sesame oil

1 ½ pounds pork shoulder, cut into strips

Himalayan salt and freshly ground black pepper, to taste

1/2 teaspoon cayenne pepper

1/2 cup shallots, roughly chopped

2 bell peppers, sliced

1/4 cup cream of onion soup

1/2 teaspoon Sriracha sauce

1 tablespoon tahini (sesame butter

1 tablespoon soy sauce

4 ounces gouda cheese, cut into small pieces

Directions:

Heat he sesame oil in a wok over a moderately high flame.

Stir-fry the pork strips for 3 to 4 minutes or until just browned on all sides. Add in the spices, shallots and bell peppers and continue to cook for a further 4 minutes.

Stir in the cream of onion soup, Sriracha, sesame butter, and soy sauce; continue to cook for to 4 minutes more.

Top with the cheese and continue to cook until the cheese has melted.

Storing

Place your stir-fry in six airtight containers or Ziploc bags; keep in your refrigerator for 3 to 4 days.

For freezing, wrap tightly with heavy-duty aluminum foil or freezer wrap. It will maintain the best quality for 2 to 3 months. Defrost in the refrigerator and reheat in your wok.

Nutrition Info: 424 Calories; 29.4g Fat; 3. Carbs; 34.2g Protein; 0.6g Fiber

Pork In Blue Cheese Sauce

Servings: 6

Cooking Time: 30 Minutes

Ingredients:

2 pounds pork center cut loin roast, boneless and cut into 6 pieces

1 tablespoon coconut aminos

6 ounces blue cheese

1/3 cup heavy cream

1/3 cup port wine

1/3 cup roasted vegetable broth, preferably homemade

1 teaspoon dried hot chile flakes

1 teaspoon dried rosemary

1 tablespoon lard

1 shallot, chopped

2 garlic cloves, chopped

Salt and freshly cracked black peppercorns, to taste

Directions:

Rub each piece of the pork with salt, black peppercorns, and rosemary.

Melt the lard in a saucepan over a moderately high flame. Sear the pork on all sides about 15 minutes; set aside.

Cook the shallot and garlic until they've softened. Add in port wine to scrape up any brown bits from the bottom.

Reduce the heat to medium-low and add in the remaining ingredients; continue to simmer until the sauce has thickened and reduced.

Storing

Divide the pork and sauce into six portions; place each portion in a separate airtight container or Ziploc bag; keep in your refrigerator for 3 to 4 days.

Freeze the pork and sauce in airtight containers or heavy-duty freezer bags. Freeze up to 4 months. Defrost in the refrigerator. Bon appétit!

Nutrition Info: 34Calories; 18.9g Fat; 1.9g Carbs; 40.3g Protein; 0.3g Fiber

Mississippi Pulled Pork

Servings: 4

Cooking Time: 6 Hours

Ingredients:

1 ½ pounds pork shoulder

1 tablespoon liquid smoke sauce

1 teaspoon chipotle powder

Au Jus gravy seasoning packet

2 onions, cut into wedges

Kosher salt and freshly ground black pepper, taste

Directions:

Mix the liquid smoke sauce, chipotle powder, Au Jus gravy seasoning packet, salt and pepper. Rub the spice mixture into the pork on all sides.

Wrap in plastic wrap and let it marinate in your refrigerator for 3 hours.

Prepare your grill for indirect heat. Place the pork butt roast on the grate over a drip pan and top with onions; cover the grill and cook for about 6 hours.

Transfer the pork to a cutting board. Now, shred the meat into bite-sized pieces using two forks.

Storing

Divide the pork between four airtight containers or Ziploc bags; keep in your refrigerator for up to 3 to 5 days.

For freezing, place the pork in airtight containers or heavy-duty freezer bags. Freeze up to 4 months. Defrost in the refrigerator. Bon appétit!

Nutrition Info: 350 Calories; 11g Fat; 5g Carbs; 53.6g Protein; 2.2g Fiber

Spicy And Cheesy Turkey Dip

Servings: 4

Cooking Time: 25 Minutes

Ingredients:

1 Fresno chili pepper, deveined and minced

1 ½ cups Ricotta cheese, creamed, 4% fat, softened

1/4 cup sour cream

1 tablespoon butter, room temperature

1 shallot, chopped

1 teaspoon garlic, pressed

1 pound ground turkey

1/2 cup goat cheese, shredded

Salt and black pepper, to taste

1 ½ cups Gruyère, shredded

Directions:

Melt the butter in a frying pan over a moderately high flame. Now, sauté the onion and garlic until they have softened.

Stir in the ground turkey and continue to cook until it is no longer pink.

Transfer the sautéed mixture to a lightly greased baking dish. Add in Ricotta, sour cream, goat cheese, salt, pepper, and chili pepper.

Top with the shredded Gruyère cheese. Bake in the preheated oven at 350 degrees F for about 20 minutes or until hot and bubbly in top.

Storing

Place your dip in an airtight container; keep in your refrigerator for up 3 to 4 days. Enjoy!

Nutrition Info: 284 Calories; 19g Fat; 3.2g Carbs; 26. Protein; 1.6g Fiber

Turkey Chorizo With Bok Choy

Servings: 4

Cooking Time: 50 Minutes

Ingredients:

4 mild turkey Chorizo, sliced

1/2 cup full-fat milk

6 ounces Gruyère cheese, preferably freshly grated

1 yellow onion, chopped

Coarse salt and ground black pepper, to taste

1 pound Bok choy, tough stem ends trimmed

1 cup cream of mushroom soup

1 tablespoon lard, room temperature

Directions:

Melt the lard in a nonstick skillet over a moderate flame; cook the Chorizo sausage for about 5 minutes, stirring occasionally to ensure even cooking; reserve.

Add in the onion, salt, pepper, Bok choy, and cream of mushroom soup. Continue to cook for 4 minutes longer or until the vegetables have softened.

Spoon the mixture into a lightly oiled casserole dish. Top with the reserved Chorizo.

In a mixing bowl, thoroughly combine the milk and cheese. Pour the cheese mixture over the sausage.

Cover with foil and bake at 36degrees F for about 35 minutes.

Storing

Cut your casserole into four portions. Place each portion in an airtight container; keep in your refrigerator for 3 to 4 days.

For freezing, wrap your portions tightly with heavy-duty aluminum foil or freezer wrap. Freeze up to 1 to 2 months. Defrost in the refrigerator. Enjoy!

Nutrition Info: 18Calories; 12g Fat; 2.6g Carbs; 9.4g Protein; 1g Fiber

Spicy Chicken Breasts

Servings: 6

Cooking Time: 30 Minutes

Ingredients:

1 ½ pounds chicken breasts

1 bell pepper, deveined and chopped

1 leek, chopped

1 tomato, pureed

2 tablespoons coriander

2 garlic cloves, minced

1 teaspoon cayenne pepper

1 teaspoon dry thyme

1/4 cup coconut aminos

Sea salt and ground black pepper, to taste

Directions:

Rub each chicken breasts with the garlic, cayenne pepper, thyme, salt and black pepper. Cook the chicken in a saucepan over medium-high heat.

Sear for about 5 minutes until golden brown on all sides.

Fold in the tomato puree and coconut aminos and bring it to a boil. Add in the pepper, leek, and coriander.

Reduce the heat to simmer. Continue to cook, partially covered, for about 20 minutes.

Storing

Place the chicken breasts in airtight containers or Ziploc bags; keep in your refrigerator for 3 to 4 days.

For freezing, place the chicken breasts in airtight containers or heavy-duty freezer bags. It will maintain the best quality for about 4 months. Defrost in the refrigerator. Bon appétit!

Nutrition Info: 239 Calories; 6g Fat; 5.5g Carbs; 34.3g Protein; 1g Fiber

Saucy Boston Butt

Servings: 8

Cooking Time: 1 Hour 20 Minutes

Ingredients:

1 tablespoon lard, room temperature

2 pounds Boston butt, cubed

Salt and freshly ground pepper

1/2 teaspoon mustard powder

A bunch of spring onions, chopped

2 garlic cloves, minced

1/2 tablespoon ground cardamom

2 tomatoes, pureed

1 bell pepper, deveined and chopped

1 jalapeno pepper, deveined and finely chopped

1/2 cup unsweetened coconut milk

2 cups chicken bone broth

Directions:

In a wok, melt the lard over moderate heat. Season the pork belly with salt, pepper and mustard powder.

Sear the pork for 8 to 10 minutes, stirring periodically to ensure even cooking; set aside, keeping it warm.

In the same wok, sauté the spring onions, garlic, and cardamom. Spoon the sautéed vegetables along with the reserved pork into the slow cooker.

Add in the remaining ingredients, cover with the lid and cook for 1 hour 10 minutes over low heat.

Storing

Divide the pork and vegetables between airtight containers or Ziploc bags; keep in your refrigerator for up to 3 to 5 days.

For freezing, place the pork and vegetables in airtight containers or heavy-duty freezer bags. Freeze up to 4 months. Defrost in the refrigerator. Bon appétit!

Nutrition Info: 369 Calories; 20.2g Fat; 2.9g Carbs; 41.3g Protein; 0.7g Fiber

Old-fashioned Goulash

Servings: 4

Cooking Time: 9 Hours 10 Minutes

Ingredients:

1 ½ pounds pork butt, chopped

1 teaspoon sweet Hungarian paprika

2 Hungarian hot peppers, deveined and minced

1 cup leeks, chopped

1 ½ tablespoons lard

1 teaspoon caraway seeds, ground

4 cups vegetable broth

2 garlic cloves, crushed

1 teaspoons cayenne pepper

2 cups tomato sauce with herbs

1 ½ pounds pork butt, chopped

1 teaspoon sweet Hungarian paprika

2 Hungarian hot peppers, deveined and minced

1 cup leeks, chopped

1 ½ tablespoons lard

1 teaspoon caraway seeds, ground

4 cups vegetable broth

2 garlic cloves, crushed

1 teaspoons cayenne pepper

2 cups tomato sauce with herbs

Directions:

Melt the lard in a heavy-bottomed pot over medium-high heat. Sear the pork for 5 to 6 minutes until just browned on all sides; set aside.

Add in the leeks and garlic; continue to cook until they have softened.

Place the reserved pork along with the sautéed mixture in your crock pot. Add in the other ingredients and stir to combine.

Cover with the lid and slow cook for 9 hours on the lowest setting.

Storing

Spoon your goulash into four airtight containers or Ziploc bags; keep in your refrigerator for up to 3 to 4 days.

For freezing, place the goulash in airtight containers. Freeze up to 4 to 6 months. Defrost in the refrigerator. Enjoy!

Nutrition Info: 456 Calories; 27g Fat; 6.7g Carbs; 32g Protein; 3.4g Fiber

Flatbread With Chicken Liver Pâté

Servings: 4

Cooking Time: 2 Hours 15 Minutes

Ingredients:

1 yellow onion, finely chopped

10 ounces chicken livers

1/2 teaspoon Mediterranean seasoning blend

4 tablespoons olive oil

1 garlic clove, minced

For Flatbread:

1 cup lukewarm water

1/2 stick butter

1/2 cup flax meal

1 ½ tablespoons psyllium husks

1 ¼ cups almond flour

Directions:

Pulse the chicken livers along with the seasoning blend, olive oil, onion and garlic in your food processor; reserve.

Mix the dry ingredients for the flatbread. Mix in all the wet ingredients. Whisk to combine well.

Let it stand at room temperature for 2 hours. Divide the dough into 8 balls and roll them out on a flat surface.

In a lightly greased pan, cook your flatbread for 1 minute on each side or until golden.

Storing

Wrap the chicken liver pate in foil before packing it into airtight containers; keep in your refrigerator for up to 7 days.

For freezing, place the chicken liver pate in airtight containers or heavy-duty freezer bags. Freeze up to 2 months. Defrost overnight in the refrigerator.

As for the keto flatbread, wrap them in foil before packing them into airtight containers; keep in your refrigerator for up to 4 days.

Bon appétit!

Nutrition Info: 395 Calories; 30.2g Fat; 3.6g Carbs; 17.9g Protein; 0.5g Fiber

Sunday Chicken With Cauliflower Salad

Servings: 2

Cooking Time: 20 Minutes

Ingredients:

1 teaspoon hot paprika

2 tablespoons fresh basil, snipped

1/2 cup mayonnaise

1 teaspoon mustard

2 teaspoons butter

2 chicken wings

1/2 cup cheddar cheese, shredded

Sea salt and ground black pepper, to taste

2 tablespoons dry sherry

1 shallot, finely minced

1/2 head of cauliflower

Directions:

Boil the cauliflower in a pot of salted water until it has softened; cut into small florets and place in a salad bowl.

Melt the butter in a saucepan over medium-high heat. Cook the chicken for about 8 minutes or until the skin is crisp and browned. Season with hot paprika salt, and black pepper.

Whisk the mayonnaise, mustard, dry sherry, and shallot and dress your salad. Top with cheddar cheese and fresh basil.

Storing

Place the chicken wings in airtight containers or Ziploc bags; keep in your refrigerator for up 3 to 4 days.

Keep the cauliflower salad in your refrigerator for up 3 days.

For freezing, place the chicken wings in airtight containers or heavy-duty freezer bags. Freeze up to 3 months. Once thawed in the refrigerator, reheat in a saucepan until thoroughly warmed.

Nutrition Info: 444 Calories; 36g Fat; 5.7g Carbs; 20.6g Protein; 4.3g Fiber

Kansas-style Meatloaf

Servings: 8

Cooking Time: 1 Hour 10 Minutes

Ingredients:

2 pounds ground pork

2 eggs, beaten

1/2 cup onions, chopped

1/2 cup marinara sauce, bottled

8 ounces Colby cheese, shredded

1 teaspoon granulated garlic

Sea salt and freshly ground black pepper, to taste

1 teaspoon lime zest

1 teaspoon mustard seeds

1/2 cup tomato puree

1 tablespoon Erythritol

Directions:

Mix the ground pork with the eggs, onions, marinara salsa, cheese, granulated garlic, salt, pepper, lime zest, and mustard seeds; mix to combine.

Press the mixture into a lightly-greased loaf pan. Mix the tomato paste with the Erythritol and spread the mixture over the top of your meatloaf.

Bake in the preheated oven at 5 degrees F for about 1 hour 10 minutes, rotating the pan halfway through the cook time.

Storing

Wrap your meatloaf tightly with heavy-duty aluminum foil or plastic wrap. Then, keep in your refrigerator for up to 3 to 4 days.

For freezing, wrap your meatloaf tightly to prevent freezer burn. Freeze up to 3 to 4 months. Defrost in the refrigerator. Bon appétit!

Nutrition Info: 318 Calories; 14. Fat; 6.2g Carbs; 39.3g Protein; 0.3g Fiber

Mexican-style Turkey Bacon Bites

Servings: 4

Cooking Time: 5 Minutes

Ingredients:

4 ounces turkey bacon, chopped

4 ounces Neufchatel cheese

1 tablespoon butter, cold

1 jalapeno pepper, deveined and minced

1 teaspoon Mexican oregano

2 tablespoons scallions, finely chopped

Directions:

Thoroughly combine all ingredients in a mixing bowl.

Roll the mixture into 8 balls.

Storing

Divide the turkey bacon bites between two airtight containers or Ziploc bags; keep in your refrigerator for up 3 to days.

Nutrition Info: 19Calories; 16.7g Fat; 2.2g Carbs; 8.8g Protein; 0.3g Fiber

Breakfast Muffins With Ground Pork

Servings: 6

Cooking Time: 25 Minutes

Ingredients:

1 stick butter

3 large eggs, lightly beaten

2 tablespoons full-fat milk

1/2 teaspoon ground cardamom

3 ½ cups almond flour

2 tablespoons flaxseed meal

1 teaspoon baking powder

2 cups ground pork

Salt and pepper, to your liking

1/2 teaspoon dried basil

Directions:

In the preheated frying pan, cook the ground pork until the juices run clear, approximately 5 minutes.

Add in the remaining ingredients and stir until well combined.

Spoon the mixture into lightly greased muffin cups. Bake in the preheated oven at 5 degrees F for about 17 minutes.

Allow your muffins to cool down before unmolding and storing.

Storing

Place your muffins in the airtight containers or Ziploc bags; keep in the refrigerator for a week.

For freezing, divide your muffins among Ziploc bags and freeze up to 3 months. Defrost in your microwave for a couple of minutes. Bon appétit!

Nutrition Info: 330 Calories; 30.3g Fat; 2.3g Carbs; 19g Protein; 1.2g Fiber

Mediterranean-style Cheesy Pork Loin

Servings: 4

Cooking Time: 25 Minutes

Ingredients:

1 pound pork loin, cut into 1-inch-thick pieces

1 teaspoon Mediterranean seasoning mix

Salt and pepper, to taste

1 onion, sliced

1 teaspoon fresh garlic, smashed

2 tablespoons black olives, pitted and sliced

2 tablespoons balsamic vinegar

1/2 cup Romano cheese, grated

2 tablespoons butter, room temperature

1 tablespoon curry paste

1 cup roasted vegetable broth

1 tablespoon oyster sauce

Directions:

In a frying pan, melt the butter over a moderately high heat. Once hot, cook the pork until browned on all sides; season with salt and black pepper and set aside.

In the pan drippings, cook the onion and garlic for 4 to 5 minutes or until they've softened.

Add in the Mediterranean seasoning mix, curry paste, and vegetable broth. Continue to cook until the sauce has thickened and reduced slightly or about 10 minutes. Add in the remaining ingredients along with the reserved pork.

Top with cheese and cook for 10 minutes longer or until cooked through.

Storing

Divide the pork loin between four airtight containers; keep in your refrigerator for 3 to 5 days.

For freezing, place the pork loin in airtight containers or heavy-duty freezer bags. Freeze up to 4 to 6 months. Defrost in the refrigerator. Enjoy!

Nutrition Info: 476 Calories; 35.3g Fat; 6.2g Carbs; 31.1g Protein; 1.4g Fiber

Oven-roasted Spare Ribs

Servings: 6

Cooking Time: 3 Hour 40 Minutes

Ingredients:

2 pounds spare ribs

1 garlic clove, minced

1 teaspoon dried marjoram

1 lime, halved

Salt and ground black pepper, to taste

Directions: Toss all ingredients in a ceramic dish.

Cover and let it refrigerate for 5 to 6 hours.

Roast the foil-wrapped ribs in the preheated oven at 275 degrees F degrees for about hours 30 minutes.

Storing

Divide the ribs into six portions. Place each portion of ribs in an airtight container; keep in your refrigerator for 3 to days.

For freezing, place the ribs in airtight containers or heavy-duty freezer bags. Freeze up to 4 to months. Defrost in the refrigerator and reheat in the preheated oven. Bon appétit!

Nutrition Info: 385 Calories; 29g Fat; 1.8g Carbs; 28.3g Protein; 0.1g Fiber

Parmesan Chicken Salad

Servings: 6

Cooking Time: 20 Minutes

Ingredients:

2 romaine hearts, leaves separated

Flaky sea salt and ground black pepper, to taste

1/4 teaspoon chili pepper flakes

1 teaspoon dried basil

1/4 cup Parmesan, finely grated

2 chicken breasts

2 Lebanese cucumbers, sliced

For the dressing:

2 large egg yolks

1 teaspoon Dijon mustard

1 tablespoon fresh lemon juice

1/4 cup olive oil

2 garlic cloves, minced

Directions:

In a grilling pan, cook the chicken breast until no longer pink or until a meat thermometer registers 5 degrees F. Slice the chicken into strips.

Storing

Place the chicken breasts in airtight containers or Ziploc bags; keep in your refrigerator for to 4 days.

For freezing, place the chicken breasts in airtight containers or heavy-duty freezer bags. It will maintain the best quality for about months. Defrost in the refrigerator.

Toss the chicken with the other ingredients. Prepare the dressing by whisking all the ingredients.

Dress the salad and enjoy! Keep the salad in your refrigerator for 3 to 5 days.

Nutrition Info: 183 Calories; 12.5g Fat; 1. Carbs; 16.3g Protein; 0.9g Fiber

Turkey Wings With Gravy

Servings: 6

Cooking Time: 6 Hours

Ingredients:

2 pounds turkey wings

1/2 teaspoon cayenne pepper

4 garlic cloves, sliced

1 large onion, chopped

Salt and pepper, to taste

1 teaspoon dried marjoram

1 tablespoon butter, room temperature

1 tablespoon Dijon mustard

For the Gravy:

1 cup double cream

Salt and black pepper, to taste

1/2 stick butter

3/4 teaspoon guar gum

Directions:

Rub the turkey wings with the Dijon mustard and tablespoon of butter. Preheat a grill pan over medium-high heat.

Sear the turkey wings for 10 minutes on all sides.

Transfer the turkey to your Crock pot; add in the garlic, onion, salt, pepper, marjoram, and cayenne pepper. Cover and cook on low setting for 6 hours.

Melt 1/2 stick of the butter in a frying pan. Add in the cream and whisk until cooked through.

Next, stir in the guar gum, salt, and black pepper along with cooking juices. Let it cook until the sauce has reduced by half.

Storing

Wrap the turkey wings in foil before packing them into airtight containers; keep in your refrigerator for up to 3 to 4 days.

For freezing, place the turkey wings in airtight containers or heavy-duty freezer bags. Freeze up to 2 to 3 months. Defrost in the refrigerator.

Keep your gravy in refrigerator for up to 2 days.

Nutrition Info: 280 Calories; 22.2g Fat; 4.3g Carbs; 15.8g Protein; 0.8g Fiber

Pork Chops With Herbs

Servings: 4

Cooking Time: 20 Minutes

Ingredients:

1 tablespoon butter

1 pound pork chops

2 rosemary sprigs, minced

1 teaspoon dried marjoram

1 teaspoon dried parsley

A bunch of spring onions, roughly chopped

1 thyme sprig, minced

1/2 teaspoon granulated garlic

1/2 teaspoon paprika, crushed

Coarse salt and ground black pepper, to taste

Directions:

Season the pork chops with the granulated garlic, paprika, salt, and black pepper.

Melt the butter in a frying pan over a moderate flame. Cook the pork chops for 6 to 8 minutes, turning them occasionally to ensure even cooking.

Add in the remaining ingredients and cook an additional 4 minutes.

Storing

Divide the pork chops into four portions; place each portion in a separate airtight container or Ziploc bag; keep in your refrigerator for 3 to 4 days.

Freeze the pork chops in airtight containers or heavy-duty freezer bags. Freeze up to 4 months. Defrost in the refrigerator. Bon appétit!

Nutrition Info: 192 Calories; 6.9g Fat; 0.9g Carbs; 29.8g Protein; 0.4g Fiber

Ground Pork Stuffed Peppers

Servings: 4

Cooking Time: 40 Minutes

Ingredients:

6 bell peppers, deveined

1 tablespoon vegetable oil

1 shallot, chopped

1 garlic clove, minced

1/2 pound ground pork

1/3 pound ground veal

1 ripe tomato, chopped

1/2 teaspoon mustard seeds

Sea salt and ground black pepper, to taste

Directions:

Parboil the peppers for 5 minutes.

Heat the vegetable oil in a frying pan that is preheated over a moderate heat. Cook the shallot and garlic for 3 to 4 minutes until they've softened.

Stir in the ground meat and cook, breaking apart with a fork, for about 6 minutes. Add the chopped tomatoes, mustard seeds, salt, and pepper.

Continue to cook for 5 minutes or until heated through. Divide the filling between the peppers and transfer them to a baking pan.

Bake in the preheated oven at 36degrees F approximately 25 minutes.

Storing

Place the peppers in airtight containers or Ziploc bags; keep in your refrigerator for up to 3 to 4 days.

For freezing, place the peppers in airtight containers or heavy-duty freezer bags. Freeze up to 2 to 3 months. Defrost in the refrigerator. Bon appétit!

Nutrition Info: 2 Calories; 20.5g Fat; 8.2g Carbs; 18.2g Protein; 1.5g Fiber

Grilled Chicken Salad With Avocado

Servings: 4

Cooking Time: 20 Minutes

Ingredients:

1/3 cup olive oil

2 chicken breasts

Sea salt and crushed red pepper flakes

2 egg yolks

1 tablespoon fresh lemon juice

1/2 teaspoon celery seeds

1 tablespoon coconut aminos

1 large-sized avocado, pitted and sliced

Directions:

Grill the chicken breasts for about 4 minutes per side. Season with salt and pepper, to taste.

Slice the grilled chicken into bite-sized strips.

To make the dressing, whisk the egg yolks, lemon juice, celery seeds, olive oil and coconut aminos in a measuring cup.

Storing

Place the chicken breasts in airtight containers or Ziploc bags; keep in your refrigerator for 3 to 4 days.

For freezing, place the chicken breasts in airtight containers or heavy-duty freezer bags. It will maintain the best quality for about 4 months. Defrost in the refrigerator.

Store dressing in your refrigerator for 3 to 4 days. Dress the salad and garnish with fresh avocado. Bon appétit!

Nutrition Info: 40Calories; 34.2g Fat; 4.8g Carbs; 22.7g Protein; 3.1g Fiber

Easy Fall-off-the-bone Ribs

Servings: 4

Cooking Time: 8 Hours

Ingredients:

1 pound baby back ribs

4 tablespoons coconut aminos

1/4 cup dry red wine

1/2 teaspoon cayenne pepper

1 garlic clove, crushed

1 teaspoon Italian herb mix

1 tablespoon butter

1 teaspoon Serrano pepper, minced

1 Italian pepper, thinly sliced

1 teaspoon grated lemon zest

Directions:

Butter the sides and bottom of your Crock pot. Place the pork and peppers on the bottom.

Add in the remaining ingredients.

Slow cook for 9 hours on Low heat setting.

Storing

Divide the baby back ribs into four portions. Place each portion of the ribs along with the peppers in an airtight container; keep in your refrigerator for 3 to days.

For freezing, place the ribs in airtight containers or heavy-duty freezer bags. Freeze up to 4 to months. Defrost in the refrigerator. Reheat in your oven at 250 degrees F until heated through.

Nutrition Info: 192 Calories; 6.9g Fat; 0.9g Carbs; 29.8g Protein; 0.5g Fiber

Brie-stuffed Meatballs

Servings: 5

Cooking Time: 25 Minutes

Ingredients:

2 eggs, beaten

1 pound ground pork

1/3 cup double cream

1 tablespoon fresh parsley

Kosher salt and ground black pepper

1 teaspoon dried rosemary

10 (1-inch cubes of brie cheese

2 tablespoons scallions, minced

2 cloves garlic, minced

Directions:

Mix all ingredients, except for the brie cheese, until everything is well incorporated.

Roll the mixture into 10 patties; place a piece of cheese in the center of each patty and roll into a ball.

Roast in the preheated oven at 0 degrees F for about 20 minutes.

Storing

Place the meatballs in airtight containers or Ziploc bags; keep in your refrigerator for up to 3 to 4 days.

Freeze the meatballs in airtight containers or heavy-duty freezer bags. Freeze up to 3 to 4 months. To defrost, slowly reheat in a saucepan. Bon appétit!

Nutrition Info: 302 Calories; 13g Fat; 1.9g Carbs; 33.4g Protein; 0.3g Fiber

Spicy And Tangy Chicken Drumsticks

Servings: 6

Cooking Time: 55 Minutes

Ingredients:

3 chicken drumsticks, cut into chunks

1/2 stick butter

2 eggs

1/4 cup hemp seeds, ground

Salt and cayenne pepper, to taste

2 tablespoons coconut aminos

3 teaspoons red wine vinegar

2 tablespoons salsa

2 cloves garlic, minced

Directions:

Rub the chicken with the butter, salt, and cayenne pepper.

Drizzle the chicken with the coconut aminos, vinegar, salsa, and garlic. Allow it to stand for 30 minutes in your refrigerator.

Whisk the eggs with the hemp seeds. Dip each chicken strip in the egg mixture. Place the chicken chunks in a parchment-lined baking pan.

Roast in the preheated oven at 390 degrees F for 25 minutes.

Storing

Divide the roasted chicken between airtight containers; keep in your refrigerator for up 3 to 4 days.

For freezing, place the roasted chicken in airtight containers or heavy-duty freezer bags. Freeze up to 3 months. Defrost in the refrigerator and reheat in a pan. Enjoy!

Nutrition Info: 420 Calories; 22g Fat; 5g Carbs; 35.3g Protein; 0.8g Fiber

Italian-style Chicken Meatballs With Parmesan

Servings: 6

Cooking Time: 20 Minutes

Ingredients:

For the Meatballs:

1 ¼ pounds chicken, ground

1 tablespoon sage leaves, chopped

1 teaspoon shallot powder

1 teaspoon porcini powder

2 garlic cloves, finely minced

1/3 teaspoon dried basil

3/4 cup Parmesan cheese, grated

2 eggs, lightly beaten

Salt and ground black pepper, to your liking

1/2 teaspoon cayenne pepper

For the sauce:

2 tomatoes, pureed

1 cup chicken consommé

2 ½ tablespoons lard, room temperature

1 onion, peeled and finely chopped

Directions:

In a mixing bowl, combine all ingredients for the meatballs. Roll the mixture into bite-sized balls.

Melt 1 tablespoon of lard in a skillet over a moderately high heat. Sear the meatballs for about 3 minutes or until they are thoroughly cooked; reserve.

Melt the remaining lard and cook the onions until tender and translucent. Add in pureed tomatoes and chicken consommé and continue to cook for 4 minutes longer.

Add in the reserved meatballs, turn the heat to simmer and continue to cook for 6 to 7 minutes.

Storing

Place the meatballs in airtight containers or Ziploc bags; keep in your refrigerator for up to 3 to 4 days.

Freeze the meatballs in airtight containers or heavy-duty freezer bags. Freeze up to 3 to 4 months. To defrost, slowly reheat in a saucepan. Bon appétit!

Nutrition Info: 252 Calories; 9.7g Fat; 5.3g Carbs; 34.2g Protein; 1.4g Fiber

SAUCES AND DRESSINGS RECIPES

Tzatziki Sauce

Servings: 2½ Cups

Cooking Time: 15 Minutes

Ingredients:

1 English cucumber

2 cups low-fat (2%) plain Greek yogurt

1 tablespoon olive oil

2 teaspoons freshly squeezed lemon juice

½ teaspoon chopped garlic

½ teaspoon kosher salt

⅛ teaspoon freshly ground black pepper

2 tablespoons chopped fresh dill

2 tablespoons chopped fresh mint

Directions:

Place a sieve over a medium bowl. Grate the cucumber, with the skin, over the sieve. Press the grated cucumber into the sieve with the flat surface of a spatula to press as much liquid out as possible.

In a separate medium bowl, place the yogurt, oil, lemon juice, garlic, salt, pepper, dill, and mint and stir to combine.

Press on the cucumber one last time, then add it to the yogurt mixture. Stir to combine. Taste and add more salt and lemon juice if necessary.

Scoop the sauce into a container and refrigerate.

STORAGE: Store the covered container in the refrigerator for up to days.

Nutrition Info: Per Serving (¼ cup): Total calories: 51; Total fat: 2g; Saturated fat: 1g; Sodium: 137mg; Carbohydrates: 3g; Fiber: <1g; Protein: 5g

Fruit Salad With Mint And Orange Blossom Water

Servings: 5

Cooking Time: 10 Minutes

Ingredients:

3 cups cantaloupe, cut into 1-inch cubes

2 cups hulled and halved strawberries

½ teaspoon orange blossom water

2 tablespoons chopped fresh mint

Directions:

In a large bowl, toss all the ingredients together.

Place 1 cup of fruit salad in each of 5 containers.

STORAGE: Store covered containers in the refrigerator for up to 5 days.

Nutrition Info: Total calories: 52; Total fat: 1g; Saturated fat: <1g; Sodium: 10mg; Carbohydrates: 12g; Fiber: 2g; Protein: 1g

Roasted Broccoli And Red Onions With Pomegranate Seeds

Servings: 5

Cooking Time: 20 Minutes

Ingredients:

1 (12-ounce) package broccoli florets (about 6 cups)

1 small red onion, thinly sliced

2 tablespoons olive oil

¼ teaspoon kosher salt

1 (5.3-ounce) container pomegranate seeds (1 cup)

Directions: Preheat the oven to 425°F and line 2 sheet pans with silicone baking mats or parchment paper.

Place the broccoli and onion on the sheet pans and toss with the oil and salt. Place the pans in the oven and roast for minutes.

After removing the pans from the oven, cool the veggies, then toss with the pomegranate seeds.

Place 1 cup of veggies in each of 5 containers.

STORAGE: Store covered containers in the refrigerator for up to days.

Nutrition Info: Total calories: 118; Total fat: ; Saturated fat: 1g; Sodium: 142mg; Carbohydrates: 12g; Fiber: 4g; Protein: 2g

White Bean And Mushroom Dip

Servings: 3 Cups

Cooking Time: 8 Minutes

Ingredients:

2 teaspoons olive oil, plus 2 tablespoons

8 ounces button or cremini mushrooms, sliced

1 teaspoon chopped garlic

1 tablespoon fresh thyme leaves

2 (15.5-ounce) cans cannellini beans, drained and rinsed

2 tablespoons plus 1 teaspoon freshly squeezed lemon juice

½ teaspoon kosher salt

Directions:

Heat 2 teaspoons of oil in a -inch skillet over medium-high heat. Once the oil is shimmering, add the mushrooms and sauté for 6 minutes. Add the garlic and thyme and continue cooking for 2 minutes.

While the mushrooms are cooking, place the beans and lemon juice, the remaining tablespoons of oil, and the salt in the bowl of a food processor. Add the mushrooms as soon as they are done cooking and blend everything until smooth. Scrape down the sides of the bowl if necessary and continue to process until smooth.

Taste and adjust the seasoning with lemon juice or salt if needed.

Scoop the dip into a container and refrigerate.

STORAGE: Store the covered container in the refrigerator for up to days. Dip can be frozen for up to 3 months.

Nutrition Info: Per Serving (½ cup): Total calories: 192; Total fat: ; Saturated fat: 1g; Sodium: 197mg; Carbohydrates: 25g; Fiber: 7g; Protein: 9g

Blueberry, Flax, And Sunflower Butter Bites

Servings: 6

Cooking Time: 10 Minutes

Ingredients:

¼ cup ground flaxseed

½ cup unsweetened sunflower butter, preferably unsalted

⅓ cup dried blueberries

2 tablespoons all-fruit blueberry preserves

Zest of 1 lemon

2 tablespoons unsalted sunflower seeds

⅓ cup rolled oats

Directions: Mix all the ingredients in a medium mixing bowl until well combined.

Form 1balls, slightly smaller than a golf ball, from the mixture and place on a plate in the freezer for about 20 minutes to firm up.

Place 2 bites in each of 6 containers and refrigerate.

STORAGE: Store covered containers in the refrigerator for up to 5 days. Bites may also be stored in the freezer for up to 3 months.

Nutrition Info: Total calories: 229; Total fat: 14g; Saturated fat: 1g; Sodium: 1mg; Carbohydrates: 26g; Fiber: 3g; Protein: 7g

Dijon Red Wine Vinaigrette

Servings: ½ Cup

Cooking Time: 5 Minutes

Ingredients:

2 teaspoons Dijon mustard

3 tablespoons red wine vinegar

1 tablespoon water

¼ teaspoon dried oregano

¼ teaspoon chopped garlic

⅛ teaspoon kosher salt

¼ cup olive oil

Directions:

Place the mustard, vinegar, water, oregano, garlic, and salt in a small bowl and whisk to combine.

Whisk in the oil, pouring it into the mustard-vinegar mixture in a thin steam.

Pour the vinaigrette into a container and refrigerate.

STORAGE: Store the covered container in the refrigerator for up to 2 weeks. Allow the vinaigrette to come to room temperature and shake before serving.

Nutrition Info: Per Serving (2 tablespoons): Total calories: 123; Total fat: 14g; Saturated fat: 2g; Sodium: 133mg; Carbohydrates: 0g; Fiber: 0g; Protein: 0g

Hummus

Servings: 1½ Cups

Cooking Time: 5 Minutes

Ingredients:

1 (15-ounce) can low-sodium chickpeas, drained and rinsed

¼ cup unsalted tahini

½ teaspoon chopped garlic

¼ cup freshly squeezed lemon juice

¼ teaspoon kosher salt

3 tablespoons olive oil

3 tablespoons cold water

Directions:

Place all the ingredients in a food processor or blender and blend until smooth.

Taste and adjust the seasonings if needed.

Scoop the hummus into a container and refrigerate.

STORAGE: Store the covered container in the refrigerator for up to 5 days.

Nutrition Info: Per Serving (¼ cup): Total calories: 192; Total fat: 13g; Saturated fat: 2g; Sodium: 109mg; Carbohydrates: 16g; Fiber: ; Protein: 5g

Candied Maple-cinnamon Walnuts

Servings: 4

Cooking Time: 15 Minutes

Ingredients:

1 cup walnut halves

½ teaspoon ground cinnamon

2 tablespoons pure maple syrup

Directions:

Preheat the oven to 325°F. Line a baking sheet with a silicone baking mat or parchment paper.

In a small bowl, mix the walnuts, cinnamon, and maple syrup until the walnuts are coated.

Pour the nuts onto the baking sheet, making sure to scrape out all the maple syrup. Bake for 15 minutes. Allow the nuts to cool completely.

Place ¼ cup of nuts in each of containers or resealable sandwich bags.

STORAGE: Store covered containers at room temperature for up to 7 days.

Nutrition Info: Total calories: 190; Total fat: 17g; Saturated fat: 2g; Sodium: 2mg; Carbohydrates: 10g; Fiber: 2g; Protein: 4g

Artichoke-olive Compote

Servings: 1⅓ Cups

Cooking Time: 15 Minutes

Ingredients:

1 (6-ounce) jar marinated artichoke hearts, chopped

⅓ cup chopped pitted green olives (8 to 9 olives)

3 tablespoons chopped fresh basil

½ teaspoon freshly squeezed lemon juice

2 teaspoons olive oil

Directions:

Place all the ingredients in a medium mixing bowl and stir to combine.

Place the compote in a container and refrigerate.

STORAGE: Store the covered container in the refrigerator for up to 7 days.

Nutrition Info: Per Serving (⅓ cup): Total calories: 8 Total fat: 7g; Saturated fat: 1g; Sodium: 350mg; Carbohydrates: 5g; Fiber: <1g; Protein: <1g

GREAT MEDITERRANEAN DIET RECIPES

Tasty Greek rice

Preparation time: 10 minutes

Cooking time: 30 minutes

Servings: 4

Ingredients:

One chopped yellow onion

1 cup parsley

1 tsp dill weed

2 cups of rice

One garlic clove

1/2 cup orzo pasta

olive oil

2 tbsp lemons juice

2 cups broth

One pinch of salt

Directions :

Wash & soak the rice (15-20) min in cold water & then drain.

Take olive oil in a pan & add onion. But first, heat the oil. It will take 3-4 minutes.

Add pasta & toss until orzo gains some color & then add rice.

Add 2 tbsp of lemon juice & broth. Now boil the liquid & bring the heat to a moderate level.

Now cover the pot & cook (20 min) until rice is cooked, i.e., the liquid is absorbed completely, and rice is tendered, then remove from stove.

For better taste, leave the pot covered & do not stir the rice (10 minutes).

Now uncover & stir with parsley & lemon zest. Now, if required, place some slices of lemon on the top for garnishing.

Now serves and enjoy.

Nutrition Info: Calories: 145 kcal Fat: 6.9 g Protein: 3.3 g Carbs: 18.3 g Fiber: 5 g

Yangchow Chinese style fried rice

Preparation time: 15 minutes

Cooking time: 20 minutes

Servings: 6

Ingredients:

6 cups cooked white rice

1 cup barbecued pork

1 tsp sugars

1 tsp ginger

Ten pieces of shrimps

3/4 cup green peas

1 tsp garlic

1 1/2 tbsp soy sauce

2 tsp salt

1/4 cup green onion

Two beaten eggs

3 tbsp cooking oil

Directions :

Heat the oil & sauté ginger-garlic together. Add the shrimps & cook (1 minute).

Pour the egg mixture & cook. Divide the cooked egg into pieces.

Add rice & soy sauce, salt & sugar, and mix with other

ingredients. Add pork, which is barbecued & cook (3 minutes). Add peas & shrimp & cook 3 minutes. Add onions and cook (2 minutes). Turn off heat & transfer to a serving plate.

Nutrition Info: Calories: 301 kcal Fat: 8 g Protein: 7 g Carbs: 49 g Fiber: 2 g

Mahi-mahi pomegranate sauce

Preparation time: 5 minutes

Cooking time: 20 minutes

Servings: 2

Ingredients:

12 oz Mahi-mahi fillets

1/2 cup balsamic vinegar

1/4 cup pomegranate juice

1 tbsp olive oil

1 tbsp squeezed lemon juice

1/2 cup pomegranate seeds

Directions : Preheat microwave up to 450 deg.

Take baking dish & lay Mahi fillets, drizzle with lemon juice & olive oil.

Bake it for 15-20 minutes

Take a pan & heat vinegar, pomegranate juice & seeds over high heat.

Bring a boil & let the sauce to reduce (20 minutes)

Spoon the fillets. Serve & enjoy.

Nutrition Info: Calories: 350 kcal Fat: 1.50 g Protein: 25 g Carbs: 45 g Fiber: 3 g

Crab stew

Preparation time: 25 minutes

Cooking time: 25 minutes

Servings: 4

Ingredients:

2 tbsp sweet paprika

1/2 cup heavy cream

6 tbsp unsalted butter

1/4 lb shrimp

1 lb lump crabmeat

2 cups steamed rice

3/4 tsp chipotle Chile powder

2 tbsp all-purpose flour

1/4 cup dry sherry

2 cups clam juice

1 cup of water

One small onion

One garlic clove

Salt and pepper

1 tbsp leaf parsley

Directions :

Melt one tbsp of butter in a pan. Add shrimp & cook at moderate heat. Now add sherry & cook for 2 minutes. Add clam juice & water. Bring a boil & simmer moderately at low heat for 10 minutes. Strain broth. Now again, melt 2 tbsp butter in the pan. Add garlic & onion & cook at moderate heat till it is softened. Add paprika & chipotle, stirring for 3 minutes. Now stir with flour. Whisk broth in the pan. Cook till it becomes smooth & then bring a boil. Simmer at low heat. Whisk till it is just thickened 5 minutes. Add cream, simmer & season with salt & pepper. Take a skillet & melt 3 tbsp butter. Now gently stir the crab & cook at moderate heat.

Toss for a few minutes' till warmed 4 minutes. Season with salt & pepper, Spoon steamed rice into the shallow bowls, Ladle shellfish sauce on rice & top with crab. Sprinkle with parsley & serve.

Nutrition Info: Calories: 827 kcal Fat: 60.7 g Protein: 37.7 g Carbs: 34.6 g Fiber: 1.9 g

280. Flavor cioppino

Preparation time: 15 minutes

Cooking time: 20 minutes

Servings: 4

Ingredients:

3 tbsp olive oil

Four chopper garlic cloves

2 tsp salt

1/2 tsp pepper

One diced onion

One sliced fennel bulb

Two celery stalks

Two diced carrots

1/2 cup Italian parsley

1 tsp red pepper

1/2 lb scallops

1 lb firm fish

1/4 cup tomatoes

1 1/2 cups dry white wine

6 cups fish stock

One bay leaf

1 lb Manila clams

1 lb mussels

Directions :

Heat oil in a heavy-bottom pot. Add onion and fennel and sauté for 5 minutes, stirring. Add the carrots, celery, and garlic and continue sautéing for five more minutes. Season with salt, pepper, and chili. Add the tomato paste and stir for one minute. Add the tomatoes and their juices to the pot, along with the wine. Let the wine reduce by half, then add the stock and bay leaves. Either chicken stock and let it a simmer. Add fish and simmer for ten minutes.

Nutrition Info: Calories: 358 kcal Fat: 19.5 g Protein: 33.7 g Carbs: 12.6 g Fiber: 2.9 g

Savory zucchini loaf

Preparation time: 25 min

Cooking time: 50-55 min

Servings: 8

Ingredients:

5 tbsp of olive oil

One small, diced zucchini.

Half cup of hazelnuts.

¾ cup of tomato (sun-dried).

Half cup milk

One cup all-purpose flour.

Three eggs

2 tsp of baking powder

2/3 cup of mozzarella cheese.

¼ cup of basil.

¼ tbsp of black pepper

¼ tbsp of sea salt

Directions :

Preheat the microwave up to 350 F

Toast hazelnuts on moderate heat in a frypan. Sauté diced zucchini on medium heat (5 min).

Place tomatoes in a bowl. For ten minutes, cover it with hot water. Drain it and place it aside. Take three eggs and whisk them in a bowl. Add milk to eggs & beat. Add flour & baking soda mix until it becomes smooth. Add 5 tbsp of olive oil & pepper. Mix it well. Add other ingredients tomatoes, basil, hazelnuts & mozzarella. Mix delicately with a spatula. Spray the pan with cooking spray & pour the batter into it. Bake for almost 45 min until toothpick comes out dry and clean. Cut it into slices & serve.

Nutrition Info: Calories: 291 kcal Fat: 21g Protein: 8g Carbs:18 g Fiber: 2g

Chilled Pea and mint soup

Prep time: 20 min

Cook time: 20-25 min

Servings: 4

Ingredients:

2 tbsp of butter

One chopped onion medium size.

Two cups of water.

Two pounds of frozen green peas.

Two cups of vegetable broth.

¼ cup of fresh mint leaves

¼ cup of fresh parsley

1 tsp of fresh lemon juice.

Half tsp cayenne.

Mint leaves for garnishing

Directions :

Melt the butter in a large pan. Add onions & cook till softened for 7 minutes.

Combine vegetable stock & water in a medium-sized saucepan. Stir in 1/2 of the water mixture in the large pan along with the onions. Increase the heat & bring to boil. Add peas & bring to a boil for one minute. Remove from stove. Add remaining water mixture with the mint, parsley & cayenne. Puree with an immersion blender in a pot till it becomes smooth. Season using lime juice. Cool until chilled. Serve in the bowls with mint leaves.

Nutrition Info: Calories: 248 kcal Fat: 7g Protein: 8g Carbs:37 g Fiber: 2g

Watermelon & cantaloupe salad

Preparation time: 10 minutes

Cooking time: 0 minute

Servings: 6

Ingredients:

¼ cup of pine nuts

2 cups of diced cantaloupe,

Six cups of diced watermelon.

5 tbsp of olive oil

2/3 cup of crumbled feta cheese.

1/4 cup of fresh mint.

¼ tsp of black pepper powder.

Directions : Toast pine nuts in a pan. Add olive oil, cantaloupe & watermelon in a bowl.

Sprinkle the cheese, mint & pepper. Mix it delicately. Chill for one hour. Serve.

Nutrition Info: Calories: 241 kcal Fat: 19g Protein: 4g Carbs: 17 g Fiber: 2g

Southern-fried okra

Preparation time: 5 min

Cooking time: 25 min

Servings: 6

Ingredients:

Half cup flour-unbleached

Half cup of cornmeal.

1/8th tsp of salt

1/4th tsp of fresh black pepper

One egg.

Two tbsp of milk

1/3rd cup of sunflower oil

3 cups of fresh okra

Directions :

Preheat the microwave up to 300 F .

Mix & whisk together the flour, salt, black pepper & cayenne in a bowl.

Beat egg & milk in a bowl. Heat sunflower oil. Dip okra pieces in the egg batter & roll in a mixture. Fry in the pan. Turn over after two min. Remove the cooked okra with a spoon & drain each batch.

Transfer 1st batch to a baking dish to keep it warm while the remaining okra is cooking.

Place the 2nd batch of the fried okra in the oven till the final batch is done.

Serve it immediately.

Nutrition Info: Calories: 213 kcal Fat: 14g Protein: 5g Carbs:20 g Fiber: 3g

Pesto Pasta with Peas and Mozzarella

Preparation time: 10 minutes

Cooking time: 0 minute

Servings: 3

Ingredients:

2 cups green peas

1 cup mozzarella balls low sodium

4 cups Boiled Penna Pasta

Pesto

2 cups fresh basil leaves

¼ tsp Garlic powder

1 tbsp Lemon juice

2 tsp zest of a lemon

1/3 cup olive oil

¼ tsp Salt

¼ tsp Pepper

Directions :

For making pesto, add all the ingredients in a blender or food processor and mix them except for olive oil. Pulse until crudely sliced. Reduce the food processor's speed or blender, slowly add olive oil to it, mix it well, and blend. Scrape down the sides of the food processor/blender to fully mix the end. Add salt &

pepper. Add mozzarella, pasta, and peas into a large bowl. Add pesto according to requirement Add pesto as desired and then mix all ingredients.

Nutrition Info: Calories: 280 kcal Fat: 14 g Protein: 11 g Carbs: 27 g Fiber: 3 g

Balsamic Roasted Green Beans

Preparation time: 5 minutes

Cooking time: 17 minutes

Servings: 1 cup

Ingredients:

1 lb Green beans

2 Chopped Garlic Cloves

1 tbsp Balsamic vinegar

1 tbsp Olive oil

⅛ tsp Salt

⅛ tsp Pepper

Directions : Preheat oven to 425°F. Mix green beans along with olive oils, pepper & salt in a large bowl. Evenly spread green beans on a foil or parchment paper-lined on a baking sheet.

Bake them for 10-12 mints in the oven until it turns light brown Spread garlic with green beans & mix well to combine. Then again, bake it for another 5 minutes till beans are warm & browned. Remove from oven & toss with balsamic vinegar.

Nutrition Info: NUTRITION: Calories: 93 kcal Fat: 5 g Protein: 4 g Carbs: 12 g Fiber: 4 g

Mac in a Flash (Macaroni and Cheese)

Preparation time: 2 minutes

Cooking time: 10 minutes

Servings: 4

Ingredients:

3 cups Water

1 cup Noodles

½ cup Grated Cheddar Cheese

1 tsp Butter

⅛ tsp dry mustard

Directions : Add noodles in boiling water, boil it for 5 to 7 minutes or until tender, and then drain the boiled noodles. Sprinkle the grated cheddar cheese on the hot noodles & mix it with butter and dry grounded mustard

Nutrition Info: Calories: 179 kcal Fat: 6 g Protein: 7 g Carbs: 23 g Fiber: 0.7 g

Costa Rican Gallo Pinto

Preparation time: 5 minutes

Cooking time: 30 minutes

Servings: 4

Ingredients:

1/3 cup dry black beans

4 tbsp Olive oil

110g Chopped Onion

2 Chopped Garlic Cloves

One chopped red bell pepper

1 tsp Cumin

1 tbsp Salsa Lizano

3 cups Cooked White rice

½ tsp black pepper

Bit of smoked paprika

¼ cup Chopped Cilantro

4 Hard-boiled eggs

Salt to taste

Directions :

Preparation of beans advance. Soak black beans in one and a half cups of water at least for 2 hrs. or overnight. Add beans in boiling water and boil them until beans tender for ten-fifteen.

Save beans along with water. Preparation for Gallo pinto. Take a large frying pan and heat the oil over medium heat. Then add sliced veggies (garlic, onion, & red pepper) to it.

Fry and stir it while frying unless or until vegies becomes soft & aromatic. After adding cumin and salsa Lozano in it, mix, then gin cook gin for two to three more minutes.

Now mix the boiled bens and its water in it and again cook for just one mint.

Combine the cooked rice & make sure that stir until rice is completely mixed with the beans.

Cover the frying pan, reduce the heat & cook again for one to two minutes, till the rice is warmed. Flavor with smoked paprika, pepper & cilantro for good flavor. Finally, add this to a bowl and decorate it with a hard-boiled egg on top.

Nutrition Info: Calories: 425 kcal Fat: 19 g Protein: 13 g Carbs: 50 g Fiber: 5 g

Cheese Quiche

Preparation time: 5 minutes

Cooking time: 45 minutes

Servings: 8

Ingredients:

4 Marginally beaten eggs

Splash of Pepper

1.5 cup milk

3 oz shredded cheddar cheese

¼ cup Chopped onion

1 tsp Parsley leaves

Pastry shell un-baked

Directions :

Preheatooven to 350°F. Mix all ingredients in a large bowl & mix it perfectly. Now add already prepared unbaked pastry shell. Bake this for forty to forty-five minutes. Cut into eight slices but cool this before baking.

Nutrition Info: Calories: 189 kcal Fat: 12 g Protein: 8 g Carbs: 11 g Fiber: 0 g

Cauliflower and Broccoli

Preparation time: 5 minutes

Cooking time: 35 minutes

Servings: 12

Ingredients:

Ten bubs of Cauliflower

1 Broccoli

3 Carrots

2 tbsp Butter or margarine

¼ Chopped onion

¼ tsp Garlic salt

½ cup Water

Directions :

Cut veggies (carrots cauliflower, & broccoli) into bite-size slices & add garlic salt, butter/margarine, & onion in it. Bring water to a boil & steam vegetable until cooked, for around 30 minutes in a very large pot.

Nutrition Info: Calories: 43 kcal Fat: 2 g Protein: 1 g Carbs: 0 g Fiber: 0 g

Pesto Pita Pizza

Preparation time: 7 minutes

Cooking time: 20 minutes

Servings: 4

Ingredients:

Homemade pesto

1 cup basil leaves

1 tbsp Chopped garlic

3 tbsp Pine nuts

1/3 cup Shredded Parmesan cheese

1 tsp Pepper

1/3 cup Olive oil

Pizza

Two pita bread

1 cup sliced mushrooms

Two plum Chopped tomatoes

¼ onion Chopped Red onions

2 tbsp balsamic glaze

Directions :

Start from preparing homemade pesto by mixing garlic, basil, Parmesan, pine nuts & pepper in a food blender, and with that, slowly add olive oil in it & then set aside.

Preheatooven to 350°F.

Spread pesto on every pitaobread.

Spread layers of tomatoes, red onion & mushrooms bread.

Bake for 15 to 20 minutes.

Take out from the oven and cool it.

Sprinkle with balsamic glaze on every pizza.

Nutrition Info: Calories: 233 kcal Fat: 12 g Protein: 1 g Carbs: 14 g Fiber: 2 g